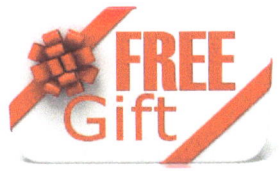

Dedication

To our three blessings that have made RicTamily complete and continue to grow together in His loving embrace.

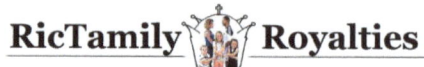

Copyright 2014-All Rights Reserved

Table of Contents

Introduction

It is unfortunate that most of the toxins that we are exposed to every day exist even in our own backyard. It is found in the air we breathe, the food we eat, the water we drink and even in the products we have inside our homes.

Even though our body possesses all the necessary tools to protect itself against harmful elements and repair itself from any damage that these elements might inflict on it, our body was not designed to handle such an exposure to toxic materials with this magnitude on a daily basis.

The main part of our body which is assigned for this huge responsibility is our liver. The liver is undoubtedly one of the most amazing organs of the body. It has the ability to deal with complex tasks and perform vital roles for our body to function as it should. But, it cannot simply handle all the work necessary to get rid of these toxic elements out of the body, and it will eventually shut down if it does not get all the help it needs.

So how do we help?

Apart from consuming only the kinds of food that strengthen and assist the liver in performing its huge list of tasks to keep the body healthy and stable, doing a liver detox will allow the body to restore its natural healing abilities by cleansing it from harmful substances. This process gives your liver a short but extremely crucial break from the dietary and lifestyle habits that may be debilitating your health. But before we delve into the program of performing a liver detox, let's get to know more about how your liver really works.

Chapter 1- What does the liver really do?

You know what a liver is; there's no doubt about that. You know it can be found in the upper right portion of your abdomen, together with the gallbladder that shares some of its functions. It is the largest, and in many ways the most complex organ of the body. You may know how it works generally – for example, it helps cleanse the body of toxins.

But, do you exactly know how it functions, what vital roles it performs for our body to stay in excellent shape, and how important it is for it to be in top shape, too?

The liver performs many functions that aid in many essential body processes, that if it is allowed to malfunction, many of these very important processes will stop and put the whole body at a serious risk.

Digestion

The liver's main contribution in the digestion process involves its production of bile, a greenish-yellow and sticky fluid, which breaks down fats so that it can be easily absorbed or eliminated by the body. Bile allows for fats to be separated into small droplets so that they can be used as nutrients by the body.

Metabolism

The liver performs very important metabolic processes especially in breaking down carbohydrates, lipids and proteins so that the body can make use of them. Carbohydrates are systematically broken down into glucose, which is stored in the form of glycogen. Hepatocytes are able to pack away and release glucose whenever the body needs it. Cholesterol and other forms of lipids are also produced by the hepatocytes to be utilized by cells throughout the body. Proteins are broken down into amino acids and undergo certain metabolic processes before they can be utilizes as energy sources.

Storage

The liver absorbs glucose from the blood that passes through the hepatic portal vein and stores it as glycogen which it can also readily release when needed by the body. The hepatocytes of the liver also absorb and store fats and other nutrients that allow the liver to keep the homeostasis of the body and to protect it from sudden spikes and drops of blood glucose levels.

Immunity

The liver also plays a vital function as an agent of the immune system of the body that helps eliminate and defend it from potentially toxic microorganisms through what is called the Kupffer cells. These cells help clean the blood passing through the hepatic portal system and the liver promptly, without having the need to launch automatic and harmful immune responses. This innate immunity system also plays an important role in liver repair.

Detoxification

The liver acts as a filtering system that monitors and automatically removes potentially toxic and harmful substances before they get to the rest of the body. Through the enzymes in hepatocytes, many of these toxins such as drugs and alcohol are converted into inactive metabolites so that they do not cause any damage to the body. The liver also eliminates some hormones out of the body's circulation to keep homeostasis and hormone levels within limits.

The liver is not only the busiest organ in the body, but also the most overworked with so many of its functions involving metabolic and chemical processes. It is said to have a variety of over five hundred tasks vital to the overall health and optimal functioning of the body.

And with toxic elimination as one of its chief and primary functions, it is also the most stressed organ in the body which is a direct result of our modern lifestyle. It is unfortunate that we do not care enough as to the kinds of foreign substances that we allow our body to consume. Although, many of these substances such as environmental pollutants, pesticides, food additives, cosmetic ingredients, etc. are beyond our control, there are more than a few that we do have direct control, and that is through our diet, such as alcohol, drugs, caffeine and many more.

If we continue to ignore and fail to make the necessary lifestyle changes, we run the risk of damaging our liver and causing it to function inefficiently.

Chapter 2- What are the symptoms of an unhealthy liver?

Detection of a liver disease at an early stage is crucial to the prevention of more severe liver problems such as cirrhosis, cancer and liver failure from developing. In order to do this, you must be aware of its symptoms so that you can seek the aid of a hepatologist, a liver specialist, before anything can get really complicated. Being able to identify accurately the signs and symptoms of liver disease will greatly increase your chances of having it treated early and successfully eliminating liver disease. A very common rule of thumb, though, is to have your liver checked at least once a year.

Below is a list of signs and symptoms of an unhealthy liver, which you can easily identify. Practically, these are symptoms you can detect on your own and without any aid from a professional doctor or hepatologist. However, if you suspect that you have liver disease based on your personal assessment according to the signs and symptoms you've learned here, it is always best to consult with your physician. Do not consider this list as completely conclusive.

Common Signs of an Unhealthy Liver

There's a myriad of liver diseases and the symptoms may tend to be specific for that particular kind of illness until the later stage of liver disease or worse, when liver failure occurs.

The initial symptoms are signs that can also happen and be caused by other problems in the body, making it rather difficult to identify liver diseases with certainty. These symptoms include nausea and vomiting, loss of appetite, diarrhea and fatigue or the feeling of being weak.

However, with the lack of immediate medication and as the complication progresses, the symptoms become more serious and require immediate care. These signs include:

Abdominal Pain

This maybe the result of having gallstones, the most common is cholesterol gallstones, which can be found usually deposited in the gallbladder and bile ducts. Pain is experienced in the upper right abdominal area of the body, and fever may occur when there is an infection in the gallbladder as a result of this

Jaundice

This is a condition wherein there is too much bilirubin in the blood stream. Bilirubin is mainly processed in the liver, therefore this excess that turns the skin, eyes and the mucus membranes in the mouth to turn yellow indicates liver damage, which can lead to liver failure if the cause is not treated.

Extreme Sleepiness

As cirrhosis, an advanced liver disease caused by a scar tissue in an attempt to perform repair of damaged tissues by the liver, develops it causes further complications. One of these complications is called hepatic encephalopathy, which stops the liver from getting the blood clear of ammonia and other nitrogenous substances, affecting cerebral functioning, such as forgetfulness, unresponsiveness, inability to concentrate and extreme sleepiness even during daytime, when it is carried to the brain.

Weight loss

A sudden decrease in weight can be caused by more than several factors. Loss of appetite, persistent vomiting, mal-absorption and increased metabolism can be some of the most obvious causes. However, there's also some evidence that points to systemic diseases such as liver diseases as one of its causes.

Chapter 3- Diseases Linked to an Unhealthy Liver

With the liver performing so many different functions for the body, and with the kind of lifestyle that we have that is sometimes debilitating, our liver becomes prone to many certain types of diseases.

Hepatitis infection

Hepatitis is a medical condition caused by the inflammation of the liver. The most common symptom is the yellow discoloration of the skin, eyes and mucus membranes. It is considered acute when it stays less than six months and chronic if it persists beyond that period. It's most common cause is viral, while the other causes are autoimmune, occurs when the body produces antibodies to fight the liver, and another type that is caused by toxins, drugs, medications and alcohol.

There are several types of viral hepatitis – Hepatitis A, B, C, D and E. Hepatitis A and E are normally contracted from the consumption of contaminated food or water, while B, C and D are through contact with contaminated bodily fluids.

The non-viral types of hepatitis can be caused by liver damage due to alcoholism, normally called "alcoholic hepatitis", or drug abuse. Autoimmune disease is caused by an error of the immune system to attack the liver thinking of it as a foreign entity that must be removed from the body.

Fatty liver

Fatty liver is the result of abnormal buildup of fats in the liver, where the body is unable to metabolize fat fast enough. There are two types of this condition, fatty liver where there is only a buildup of fat and non-alcoholic steatohepatitis which there is a buildup of fat and liver cell damage.

The most common cause of fatty liver is alcoholism, wherein almost every alcoholic has fatty liver disease. Toxins, some particular medications and some metabolic disorders cause fatty liver disease. It has also been linked to obesity, high blood and type 2 diabetes, especially for those who aren't alcoholics. It is important to note though that a high-fat diet does not always result in fatty liver disease.

Cirrhosis

This type of condition occurs and results as a complication when the liver is exposed to a liver disease for a long period of time which involves severe and irreversible scarring and loss of liver cells. Its most common causes are Hepatitis B and C and alcohol abuse.

Cirrhosis develops when the liver fails to regenerate and repair damaged cells. When this happens, the liver shrinks and hardens, which makes it difficult for the nutrient-rich blood to pass and flow into the liver. Cirrhosis of the liver can lead to a number of very serious complications, such as edemas, severe bleeding, hepatorenal syndrome, and even liver cancer.

Liver Cancer

This is a severe condition wherein liver cells become abnormal. They can grow out of control, typical of a cancer cell that destroys the organ's cells and interferes with its ability to function properly. There are many types of liver cancer, but they can be generalizes into primary and secondary or metastatic liver cancer.

Primary liver cancer begins inside the liver while secondary or metastatic liver cancer originates from the other organs of the body. Hepatocellular carcinoma is the most known primary liver cancer. Other types are cholangiosarcoma, hemangiosarcoma and hepatoblastoma.

On the other hand, the most common metastatic or secondary cancers that can spread to the liver are cancers of the colon, breast, kidney, bladder, ovary, stomach, pancreas, lungs and the uterus. Sometimes, these tumors do not have apparent symptoms, but swelling in the abdomen or jaundice can be a good indicator that cancer has affected the liver.

Chapter 4- The Most Common Elements that Harm the Liver

I don't think the importance of our liver can be over-stressed enough. It serves as the primary filter of our body that keeps us free from toxins and other harmful elements. It regulates stores, synthesizes and breaks down complex and different substances in the body creating balance and allows the body to consistently perform hundreds of separate bodily functions.

In fact, many medical and health practitioners even believe that an unhealthy liver is usually the root cause of many diseases and most serious health problems of the body. Conversely, when we are able to maintain a healthy and well-functioning liver, we avoid running the risk of getting seriously ill. It is imperative therefore for us to stay away from things that may harm our liver and cause it to be unhealthy.

So, what harms the liver?

High-protein diet

The liver metabolizes proteins into simpler compounds, so that they become readily absorbed by the body. This metabolic process is especially taxing on the liver, which means that the higher the consumption of protein, the higher the stress level on the liver becomes.

Too Much Simple Carbs

Excess simple carbs are converted and stored in the liver as fat. The more there is stored fat in the liver, the more difficult it is for the liver to perform many of its functions normally.

Overeating

Regularly eating too much food or more frequently than what your body needs to nourish and sustain it severely affects health. Doing so leaves a huge amount of undigested food in the intestinal tract that becomes a source of toxic substances. This can cause for the lymphatic system to congest and the blood to thicken which is overtaxing to the liver and other excretory organs.

Rapid Weight Loss

It is true that there are significant benefits when you lose excess weight, especially around your waist, such as normal blood pressure and cholesterol and sugar levels, but it also presents some risk. When you are trying to lose weight rapidly through some diet, namely low-fat diets that encourage you to reduce calorie intake, your tendency to develop gallstones in your liver and gallbladder also increases.

Pharmaceutical Drugs

All drugs we take for specific reasons go through the liver because they are toxic by nature and needs detoxification by the liver. Regular intake of maintenance medications will have long-term negative effects on the liver that could impair many of its functions.

Alcohol Abuse

The liver tissues can be inflamed by drinking too much alcohol. Inflammation of the liver can lead to even worse conditions such as cirrhosis especially if it persists for a long period of time.

Toxins in the environment

The air that we breathe and the food that we eat contribute to the added toxins that our liver has to purify and refine. It is unfortunate that as our world gets so modern, it also has produced more than too many pollutants that greatly affect our health. It has also caused us to adapt unhealthy lifestyles such as spending more time on doing activities that requires less and less physical energy and consume processed foods just because they are easily accessible.

Lack of exercise

Because of spending more time at work and less time in doing more physical activities, the liver is forced to eliminate toxins that should be eliminated from the body through perspiration, for example, that should be done by the skin.

Chapter 5- Why is It Important to Have a Liver Detox?

You have just learned about the many factors that harm the liver and reasons that cause liver disease. Many of these effects can be reversible and can be treated before they result in severe complications such as hepatitis, fatty liver, cirrhosis and even liver cancer.

Also, every day our bodies are exposed to many toxins from the things that surround us – from the pollutants in the air, food additives in our processed foods, chemicals in our drinking water to the synthetic ingredients in our personal care products, medications and home products. Literally, our bodies are beset by different kinds of toxins on a daily basis. According to the CDC, Center for Disease Control and Prevention, your body may contain at least 212 kinds of chemicals.

With that said, it has now even become more imperative and crucial to undergo liver detoxing or cleansing at least two to three times a year. Here are extremely important reasons why you should do a liver detox:

- You eat a diet that is largely composed of processed foods, high in sugar and unhealthful fats, has food additives that are highly refined, and foods that contain artificial sweeteners and caffeine.
- A detox can help your body eliminate many of these toxins naturally while also allowing your body to repair organs and tissues, and gives it a chance to rest.
- A detox can help improve skin problems, relieve pain and digestion problems, and boost energy levels while supporting and promoting the body's innate healing ability.
- A detox can help enhance the body's natural processes in eliminating chemicals from sweat, urine and feces.
- A detox can help your liver function properly by making sure that your diet has the necessary nutrients your body needs.

Chapter 6- Benefits of Liver Detox

Now that you are fully aware of the vital functions of your liver and how important it is to keep it in top shape, let us delve into the many benefits that you can expect from the liver detox program.

Boosts Immune System

Cleansing the liver and detoxing the body allows many of your organs to function optimally the way they should. It is said that lymphocytes comprise 25 percent of the cells in the liver, and with a healthy liver, this gives you a very efficient line of defense against diseases that manage to pass through the digestive tract. A healthy liver also allows for a better absorption of nutrients needed by the body which gives your immune system the necessary boost, which helps to ensure a healthy proliferation of immune cells that fight off diseases.

Makes Skin Healthier

Most skin disorders such as acne, discoloration or irregular texture are a result of poor waste elimination of the body. Other signs of this backlog of waste can be accelerated aging such as wrinkles, loss of collagen and decreased elasticity of the skin. When liver cleansing is performed, the removal of wastes and toxins in the body results in the sufficient formation of collagen that keeps the skin tone and texture healthier. This may also help eliminate and treat acne which results in clearer and smoother skin as you complete your detox program.

Improves Digestion

The liver is an accessory in the digestion process. It produces bile, stored in the gallbladder, which plays an important role in breaking down fats to be easily absorbed and utilized by the body. Essentially, a healthy liver promotes good digestion wherein the food we eat is broken down for its nutrients, the nutrients are easily absorbed, distributed and metabolized efficiently by the cells in the body, and the waste by-products in the process of breaking down food are fully eliminated.

Through liver cleanse and detox all these processes are properly maintained by keeping the liver healthy and functioning properly. With an improved digestion, the positive impact in your overall health cannot be overvalued.

Controls Blood Sugar

The liver helps in maintaining the circulating blood sugar levels steady and constant. It stores sugar as glycogen and releases it whenever the body needs it. Liver detox helps ensure that the liver is able to stay in top shape in order to manage blood sugar and keep it balanced at all times. Failure to do so can result in many kinds of complication that an unbalanced level of sugar can cause.

Clears the Mind

Removing damaging substances from your blood is one of the chief duties of the liver. When the liver is not healthy and does not properly function, it can negatively affect the entire body, as well as the brain. "Brain fog" is used to describe this feeling of mental fogginess, which includes forgetfulness, confusion and inability to concentrate. This is usually experienced by those who suffer from Hepatitis C or cirrhosis, a condition that affects the liver.

With liver detoxing and cleansing, many have reported that they lost that sense of fogginess and are able to think clearly during and after a liver cleansing program as compared to a state when they are not on it.

Gives You More Energy

After undergoing liver detox, many followers of the program say that they feel more energetic and enthusiastic throughout the day. This should make sense because one of the symptoms of liver disease is fatigue and feeling weak. Going through a liver detox program should help in restoring your liver into its healthier and better state. Also, liver detox programs involve modification in your diet, replacing fatty foods with fruits and vegetables that give you a natural energy boost.

Frees You from Pain

When the body experiences some problems and some parts are malfunctioning, pain is usually and normally one of the sensations that you feel. This signals the body that something needs to be corrected. It is often the proper immune system response to such a malfunction. When the pain goes away naturally, it means that the body has regained its balanced state. However, there are cases when the pain persists, which means that the root problem has not been removed yet.

Performing a liver detox can help eliminate pain from the body. When the liver is healthy and is not congested by large amounts of toxins, the vital body processes such as digestion, metabolism and elimination of wastes are efficiently performed; as a result, your immune system is able to heal any malfunction in the body successfully and naturally.

Chapter 7- How to Liver Detox – The Essential Steps

Performing detoxification of the liver must be done in a process that allows for each of the organs involved such as the kidneys and intestines working in synergy with each other. They must also be prepared for the added toxins that the liver may dump on them when you start detoxifying your liver. Therefore, it is vital that a colon and kidney detox is done first before the liver detox.

With this understanding, we will establish that a complete and better liver detox is a three-phase program that is composed of Colon Detox as Phase 1, Kidney Detox as Phase 2 and Liver Detox as Phase 3. You will have to go through each phase in the right order in order to maximize its potential holistic benefits.

Phase One – Colon Detox

Colon detox is considered to be the foundation of liver detox or liver cleansing. This is believed to be so, simply because if your intestinal tract is "clogged", many of the toxins and wastes that your kidney is going to dump on the colon will be pushed back into the bloodstream, which can actually make you ill.

To start with your colon detox, here are a few steps:

Change your diet by adding more fruit, vegetable and fiber-rich foods into your new daily meal intake, while at the same time trying to lessen your consumption of fast and processed foods.

Use supplements that aid or promotes colon cleansing. These supplements may include laxative, enemas and strong herbal teas. It is best that these supplements are used on a daily basis giving you more advantage and maximized effectiveness.

The last step is a little bit uncomfortable, which involves a colon therapist to perform what is called a colon irrigation process. The colon therapist inserts a tube and pumps water or some liquid into your rectum. The therapist massages your abdomen to push out the water and other wastes from your colon. The therapist then repeats the process to entirely cleanse the colon.

Phase Two – Kidney Detox

We know that our kidneys' primary function is to eliminate wastes out from the body, aside from maintaining balance in your body and regulating blood pressure. This is already enough reason for us to help it function optimally; thus, the kidney detox.

To perform this program, you will need to modify your diet. Eat more fruit and vegetables, especially the ones with high potassium such as bananas, apricots, kiwis and prunes.

Drink a lot of clean and natural water which helps to filter more toxins out of the body through urine. A good indicator of a clean filtering system would be passing much clearer and less smelly urine.

As part of modifying your diet to detox your kidneys, you must avoid the consumption of caffeine, chocolate, processed foods and alcohol. Also, avoid high-protein foods.

Phase Three – Liver Detox in 5 Days

It is assumed that you have already done colon and kidney detox first before performing this 5-day liver detox program. We would like to make sure that you do not experience any complications because you skipped the previous phases that are prerequisite to this phase.

It is very important to note that this liver detox program must be done in 5 days straight on an empty stomach. The first thing you need to do upon rising early in the morning is to drink a glass of water.

Day 1

Prepare a fresh squeezed apple juice of grape juice, a lemon, one clove of garlic (add one clove each day), one tablespoon of oil (add one tablespoon), and a piece of ginger with at least 8 oz of pure water in a blender. Mix and blend. Drink the concoction you just made, finishing it all down, followed by a fresh juice chaser to clear your mouth.

Fifteen to twenty minutes after drinking your first juice formula, drink at least two cups of liver detox tea (you can choose from any products readily available to you). This tea helps in the flushing process and eases any discomfort. They key ingredient for this tea drink is the dandelion root; although other herb ingredients that the tea includes are also enormously beneficial to your kidneys.

Liver Detox Tea

To prepare for your liver detox tea, you will need to fill a pot with four to five tablespoons of the tea the night before to let it soak overnight. Let is simmer for at least twenty minutes in the morning before drinking. Do the same every day.

For lunch, you can drink more juice or have some raw vegetable salad. Only make sure to prepare your own salad dressing. Use fresh olive oil, apple cider vinegar and any other fresh herbs and spices of your choice.

For dinner, eat fresh fruit or vegetables or drink only fruit juices or fruit smoothies.

Juicing Recipes

You may use any combination of the following fruit or vegetables such as an apple, a stick of celery, ginger (one-half piece) and enough carrots to make 20 – 25 oz of juice.

Days 2 – 4

Do the same preparations as the ones on Day 1. Drink the liver detox tea and as much diluted juices as you can throughout the day. Another drink to add though is to consume a lot of potassium broth. Here's how to prepare your potassium broth:

Potassium Broth Recipe

Simmer the potato skins (from 4 large potatoes), carrots (4 large carrots with skin), celery (2 sticks), beets (3 whole pieces), onions (peeled and sliced) and garlic (50 cloves) for at least an hour in a covered pot using clean water. When done, strain the vegetables and let the broth cool down and then drink it. Refrigerate what's left in glass containers so you can use it over the next few days.

Note: All the vegetables used must be organically produced.

Day 5

Simply repeat preparations from Day 1.

To complete the program, you must integrate a moderate exercise every day. Doing so will make you feel a whole lot more active and will get things moving.

Now, some people experienced a little discomfort and went through some "healing crisis". If you experience the same, this should not deter you from completing the detox program. Some of these symptoms could be feeling fatigue, nauseous, feverish or even having skin rashes or diarrhea. Fortunately, for most people, the experience of going through the detox program has been greatly rewarding and beneficial.

Chapter 8- Foods that Detox the Liver

The liver is responsible for processing almost everything that gets into the body through our diet. This includes the breaking down of proteins, carbohydrates and fats that our body uses as fuel to fulfill many of its functions for life and health to continue to flourish.

It is only imperative that we support our liver by sometimes giving it the break it needs to be able to rest and heal. This we can do by taking control of the kinds of food that we stuff ourselves. If we consciously choose to eat natural and healthy foods and avoid those that are processed and contain harmful ingredients, our liver should get enough help by reducing the toxins that we most of the time carelessly feed it.

Here are some of the most toxic foods that we should avoid:

- Highly processed and refined foods
- Foods high in trans-fat
- Foods high in sugar content

Conversely, here are foods that you should consume more to help the liver especially during the detox program. These include:

- Foods rich in vitamins and minerals, particularly vitamin A in carrots and sweet potatoes.
- Cruciferous vegetables such as broccoli, kale, collard greens, cauliflower, and cabbage.
- Foods rich in vitamin E such as spinach, olive oil, mustard greens, avocados, papaya, sunflower seeds, almonds and pumpkin. These foods help the liver to clean itself.
- Fruit such as oranges, grapefruits, strawberries, limes and others that are loaded with vitamin C. Vegetables rich in vitamin C such as broccoli, cauliflower, bell pepper, parsley and many others should also be included in your diet.
- Foods that are rich in Selenium like tuna, cod, salmon, shrimp, turkey, mushrooms, mustard seeds, nuts and garlic are also great sources of detoxifying ingredients that should assist the liver.

What we do on a regular basis makes the biggest difference in having better health, not the ones we can only afford to do occasionally. Therefore, we must make it a habit to incorporate many of the foods mentioned above that promote better health and assist the liver in achieving optimal performance.

Chapter 9- Tips to Keep a Healthy Liver and Healthier You

Do a liver cleanse two times a year.

Having your liver cleansed regularly is an important aspect in maintaining health and allowing your body to perform all of its functions more efficiently. There are far greater benefits such as better mental clarity, higher boost of energy, better immune system, more effective anti-aging, etc. that you can take advantage of when you do liver detox that makes it really absurd not to do it at all.

Eat a healthy diet.

A healthy diet includes the right amount of carbohydrates, fat, protein, vitamins, mineral and water. This is the key to maintaining energy, stamina, strength and a healthy immune system.

Eat only when you are hungry.

It is common among us to eat and grab some snacks when we are bored or have nothing better to do. This must be controlled in order to avoid stuffing yourself with unnecessary calories and toxins present in processed drinks and junk foods.

Drink ionized water frequently.

There are at least three very important benefits to drinking ionized water. One, it is an antioxidant, which means it helps you get rid of the free radicals in your body. Two, since it is alkaline it balances the pH levels of your body. And three, it is more hydrating than tap water or the water that we normally use.

Cut down on alcohol.

Cutting down on alcohol and maintaining your consumption within the guidelines will help you feel greater and enjoy benefits better concentration, you may lose weight; reduce serious side effects of alcohol, and many other benefits. It is best to drink within the allowed 3 – 4 units of alcohol daily plus days with no alcohol intake.

Avoid eating large meals.

Eating more than what your body needs can lead to excessive weight gain. It is best to consume food only until you have satisfied your hunger. Do not skip meals as well so that you avoid making up for them later, which is usually the case of stuffing a lot of food at one time. Also avoid eating before going to bed.

Avoid eating fatty food.

Fatty foods such as ice cream, French fries, cheeseburgers, etc. are loaded with unhealthy fat, sugar and salt. Do your best to replace them with healthier food that can at least provide you with the nutrients you need and keep you from consuming the unnecessary. Eat more fruit and vegetables, instead.

Avoid eating refined carbs.

These types of carbs such as white bread, white rice, etc. have mostly lost their fiber and nutritional value during the refining process, which make them virtually less useful to the body. It is far better to have whole grains, fruit, vegetables and beans in our diet.

Get enough sleep.

Getting enough sleep does not only make you feel better, more energetic and have more positive mood, but it also helps you to focus and concentrate better allowing you to have better performance at work. You will also experience being better at remembering things. Other noted benefits are a longer life, better health restoration, and even being more creative.

Avoid overworking.

It is important to avoid being burned out because of working too much. The negative effects of this are getting easily tired, stressed and losing the ability to focus and concentrate. In fact, it decreases your creativity and productivity. Spending too much time at work can also put a strain on your relationships which is always not a good thing.

Exercise regularly.

Most people nowadays have more sedentary lifestyles, spending more time in an office chair or on the couch when at home. It is always best to have some time to stand and do a little workout. Taking brisk walks outside the house or cycling around the neighborhood can help you stay active and relax while stretching some of those muscles.

Chapter 10- Frequently Asked Questions

1. Is it a waste of time to do this detox if you're a heavy drinker?

It will never be a waste of time to do the detox if you're a heavy drinker. If fact, it is necessary because it can provide the help you need to repair much of the damage on your liver by your heavy drinking. But, if you can't stop yourself from drinking even while on detox, you will probably need to learn to have enough self-control in order for this to work for you.

2. Is it okay for pregnant women to do the liver cleanse?

The liver detox has no known side effects, but it would be much safer to postpone it at least six weeks after giving birth.

3. Is there an alternative to apple juice if I cannot tolerate it?

Apple juice has the best properties for a more effective liver detox. Try to drink it very slowly and in very small amounts, and watering it down. But, if it proves really difficult for you to tolerate it, you can substitute it with 1,500 to 2,000 mg malic acid powder dissolved in two glasses of water.

4. Is it better to avoid the liver detox during my menstrual period?

Menstruating is already a form of body cleansing, which means performing the liver detox will make you cleanse from different ends. Although this is good, it will be more comfortable for women to cleanse before or after their monthly menstrual cycles.

5. Is old age an obstacle to achieving good results from the liver detox?

Old age will never be an obstacle to benefiting from the liver detox. In fact, many elderly who have gone through the program have reported that they felt greater and more energetic. The liver detox might even help improve their physical and mental state and restore them back to better health. It can also improve their bodies' ability to absorb nutrients from food and maximize the benefits from their medications or maintenance drugs.

6. Is it okay to continue taking food supplements while doing the liver cleanse?

It is best to avoid taking any food supplements during the liver detox because they will only be flushed out and become wasted.

7. Is it normal to feel very energetic in some days and very tired in others during the detox?

It is possible to have different kinds of energy levels while detoxing. Each of us can have a different reaction to it. But what has been commonly reported is a sense of clarity in thinking, better concentration and sharper senses (vision and smell).

8. Are there other symptoms I should expect?

Your body might react to the liver detox in different ways. Some of these reactions include joint or muscle pain, diarrhea, headache, fatigue, nausea, inability to sleep, mild fever, frequent urination, or skin rashes that may be perceived as an allergic reaction. You must note that if you have these reactions, it means that you are going through a "healing crisis" and should not prematurely stop the process of liver detoxing or cleansing.

9. Is it also possible to not notice anything unusual during the liver detox?

Yes. This could mean that your liver was not that toxic. But it could also mean that you only went through some partial release that's why nothing was noticeable. You may benefit from another set of the liver detox program, making at least two detoxes in a year.

10. What to do if I don't make it through the five days?

If you're feeling uncomfortable and many of the reactions unbearable at this time, you can stop. It is always possible to go back to the detox program anytime you are already feeling better or more prepared to go through the entire program.

11. Is it okay to start consuming coffee again after detoxing?

You can basically do anything after the liver detox. Drinking coffee is fine as long as you can keep it down to at least one cup a day.

12. Are there any specific rules to be followed during the first few days' right after the liver detox?

It is best to consume the cleanest and healthiest food especially in the first few days' right after the detox. Make sure that you eat fibrous food so that you avoid getting constipated when you start eating again. Raw foods such as salads are highly recommended.

13. Is it okay to leave the garlic out because I'm finding it hard to take the formula in for my liver detox?

Garlic is highly recommended for its properties that help eliminate parasites and clean the liver effectively. But if you can't really handle it, it will be okay to do the detox without it.

Medical Disclaimer

Please Check Out the Other Books by

RicTamily Royalties:

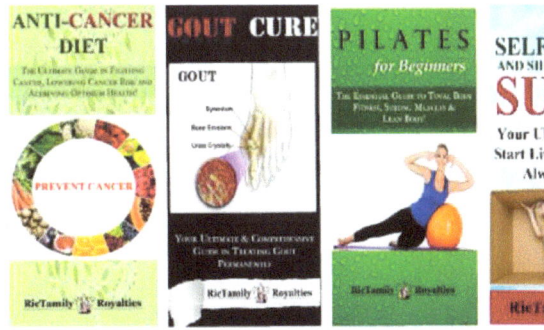

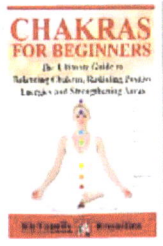
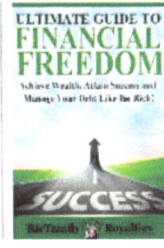
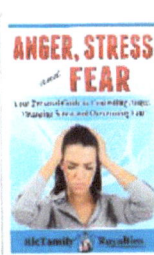
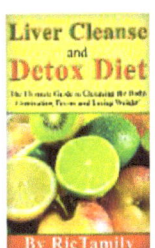

Please Leave a Review

If you enjoyed this book, we would really appreciate it if you could leave us a positive REVIEW

P.S. You can CLICK HERE to go directly to the book page and leave your review and/or purchase our other books above. Alternately, you can copy and paste this address into your browser --- http://amzn.to/1wCj3OE

THE END